Coping with
EAR PROBLE

DAVID L. COWAN

With a Foreword by
TERRY SCOTT

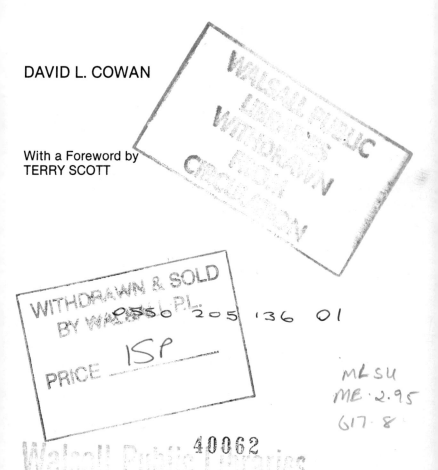

Chambers

Published by W & R Chambers Ltd Edinburgh

Illustrated by R.A. Yorston

ISBN 0 550 20513 6

British Library Cataloguing in Publication Data

Cowan, David L.
    Coping with ear problems.
    1. Hearing disorders
    I. Title
    617.8   PR290
    ISBN 0-550-20513-6

Printed in Great Britain by
Butler & Tanner Ltd, Frome and London

Contents

Foreword

There are three 'deafies' in our family—myself and two of our four daughters.

When I was at school I was nothing if not consistent... consistently at the bottom of the class, that is. They thought I was stupid, but I suspect I was lazy, and deaf. Happily there is more awareness in schools nowadays of the possibility of hearing-impairment, but my daughters will tell you how easy it is to acquire the 'thicko' label in social situations. New acquaintances will note the incomprehension, the lack of expected response, and make a quick diagnosis: 'She's not very bright, is she?' In fact, they are both quite bright enough, thank you; too bright for me sometimes! Sarah is an actress, and teaches mime and signing to children, both deaf and hearing. Ally is in her third year at college, and already disagrees with everything her father says, which only goes to show she's learning a great deal.

To go back to the 'dim and daft' label. The problem arises because there's absolutely nothing to see, especially if you're a girl, and use your hair to hide your hearing aids. Blindness is (usually) visible. Deafness is not. Some people try really hard to help. They shout. Unfortunately, shouting isn't the solution. Added to which to it makes one feel such a twit. Clarity of speech is much more helpful. It's all a question of knowing the facts.

Now, there are ear problems of many kinds—and many different types of deafness... Good heavens, for a moment there I was going to write a book about it. But I don't need to, thank goodness... Here it is.

Terry Scott
Godalming, 1986

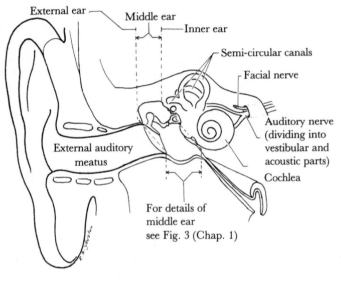

Fig. 1 The main parts of the ear.

1. How The Ear Works

The ear is a very important organ in the body. Like any other organ in the body it can go wrong and anyone who has ever suffered acute earache or deafness will know how miserable this can make one's life.

Before discussing how we can cope with various problems, it is important to have some knowledge of how the ear works. The ear has two quite distinct functions—hearing and balance—and these will be considered separately.

Anatomy of the Ear

The ear, from an anatomical point of view, consists of three distinct parts. The outer part (*external ear*) is made up by *the pinna* (the part on the outside) and *the ear canal* or external auditory meatus. The pinna has some function in collecting sound waves and you know how granny will cup her hand behind her ear to help her hear. The ear canal is not straight and this is a help as it will often prevent sharp objects going in too far and damaging the deeper structures. The canal is arched and the outer one-third is made of cartilage (like the pinna) while the inner two-thirds are bony. The whole canal is lined with skin which has many sensitive nerve endings—that is why it is very painful if your ear is ever damaged. Wax-producing glands (ceruminous glands) are present only in the outer one-third of the canal. Wax helps to lubricate the skin and also to protect the ear from dust and other foreign objects. Although wax is brown in colour it is not dirty. There is a natural movement of the skin of the ear canal *out* the way and this will bring wax out of the ear. It is not necessary to poke cotton buds or tissue paper into the ear to clean it as nature does this for us by bringing wax to the outer part of the ear. In fact, poking things into the ear is wrong as this will tend to block the canal completely. The old adage that you should never put anything smaller than your elbow in your ear is a good one.

The ear canal conducts the sound waves from the outside to *the ear drum* or *tympanic membrane* which lies 1.5 inches or 3 cm from the outer end of the canal. The ear drum is made of three very thin layers, one of which is elastic tissue, so it acts rather like the surface of a drum. When the sound waves strike the drum this will move and initiate the process of conducting the sound from the outside to the sensitive inner ear. The ear drum is very thin and can break down or perforate either by direct damage or as a result of infection. This will obviously produce some deafness

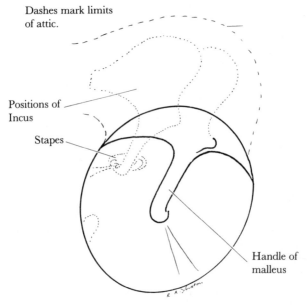

Fig. 2 View of the ear drum (through an otoscope)

because sound waves will fail to produce the normal resonant movement of the ear drum.

The ear drum protects the ear canal from the next part of the organ which is called *the middle ear*. The middle ear is a space containing air and three little bones called *ossicles*. The middle ear space is connected with the outside world by a tube which runs from the middle ear to the back of the nose on each side.

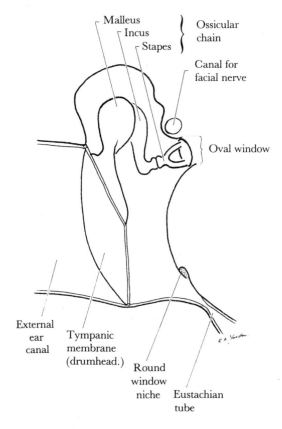

Fig. 3 The middle ear

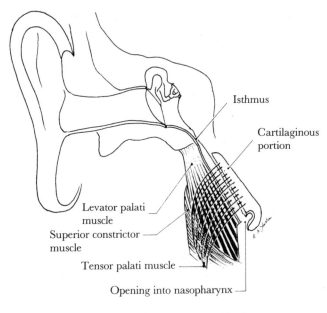

Isthmus

Cartilaginous portion

Levator palati muscle

Superior constrictor muscle

Tensor palati muscle

Opening into nasopharynx

Fig. 4 The Eustachian (pharyngo-tympanic) tube

This tube is called *the Eustachian tube* or pharyngo-tympanic tube, and it is important as it allows the pressure in the middle ear to be the same as that of the atmosphere. You all know that, if you fly when you have a cold and your Eustachian tube is blocked, you can get a very sore ear as the pressure in the middle ear is different from that in the aeroplane. This also applies to divers and they are never allowed to dive if they have a cold. The muscles that open the Eustachian tube come from the palate and that is why swallowing or sucking a sweet at take-off will help to open the tube and equalise the pressures.

The ossicles are three in number and are called *the malleus* (or hammer), *the incus* (or anvil) and *the stapes* (or stirrup). The malleus is attached to the ear drum and the ossicles conduct the sound waves from the ear drum to the sensitive hearing part of the inner ear which is called *the cochlea*. The ossicles articulate with each other and act on the lever principle to amplify the sound waves as they are transmitted through the middle ear. The ossicles are unlike any other bones in the body as they are at their full adult size when we are born.

The next and very sensitive part of the ear is *the inner ear* or *cochlea*. This is bony, shell-shaped like a snail and contains fluid and many thousands of very sensitive nerve endings. The sound waves are conducted from the ear drum by the ossicles to the inner ear. The fluid in the inner ear moves in response to the waves and the nerve endings convert this into electrical impulses which pass to the hearing centres in the brain where they are perceived as sound.

This is a simplified description of how the hearing part of the ear works—think of it like a model. It is a very sensitive organ and any of the various component parts can break down. We can be born with absent or abnormal parts. The parts can be damaged by injuries or infection and finally, of course, the parts can begin to wear out as we get older. If any of these things happen we will become deaf.

As already mentioned, the inner ear has a quite separate unrelated function which is concerned with maintaining our balance. As well as the snail (or cochlea) there are three bony semicircular canals which are all at right angles to each other.

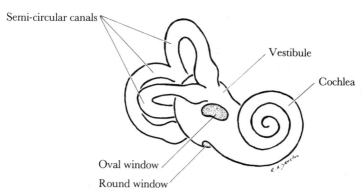

Fig. 5 The Bony labyrinth

These make up *the labyrinth*, and an inner ear infection or labyrinthitis will cause dizziness. Our ability to remain steady, walk in a straight line, etc is controlled by a variety of different mechanisms which are complex and outwith the scope of a book like this. The labyrinthine causes of dizziness are discussed in Chapter 9.

2. Pain In The Ear

The medical term for pain in the ear is *otalgia*. Most of us at some time or other have suffered from this and it can be the most excruciating discomfort which is even more distressing in childhood when it is often experienced.

Acute Otitis Media

By far the commonest cause of earache in children is acute otitis media. This is an acute infection in the middle ear which usually (but not always) occurs in association with a cold or other upper respiratory infection. The pain is due to the build up of infected fluid in the middle ear space. The Eustachian tube blocks so that the fluid cannot escape and the ear drum becomes red and bulges due to the infected fluid. The pain comes from the fact that the ear drum, which has many very sensitive nerve endings, is stretched and that is why anaesthetic ear drops will sometimes reduce the severity of the pain although they will not cure it. The pain most commonly 'comes to a head' during the night. The reason for this is not just 'Sod's law' but when we are warm in bed at night and lying down, the blood supply to the ear increases and produces the acute pain which is so common.

There is no magic treatment to immediately cure the acute pain. If the pressure becomes so great that the ear drum bursts then the pain will be immediately relieved and the ear will discharge infected fluid. In the days before antibiotics the treatment was to incise the drum and release the fluid but the vast majority of acute otitis media attacks will now settle within 24-36 hours with antibiotic medicine (or pills). Pain killers by mouth will help to deaden the pain in the meantime. Some people also advocate decongestant medicine and/or nose drops and this will certainly do no harm although will not usually produce a cure on their own. It is very important that the *full* course of antibiotic prescribed by the doctor is taken (even although the pain has gone) to prevent a recurrence of the same infection.

Recurrent attacks

An acute attack such as this is obviously a very distressing occasion for both parents and child and there is no doubt that some children are more prone to recurrent attacks than others. If the attacks are recurrent then each one must be treated with a full course of antibiotics. Parents become understandably concerned if their children require repeated courses of antibiotics and although in itself this is not a serious situation, it may be that there is some underlying treatable condition in the throat, nose or sinuses which is 'triggering off' the infections and usually it is worth seeking the advice of an ear, nose and throat specialist if attacks recur.

The other fear that people have is that their child's hearing may be damaged permanently by one or other of the infections. Although the child will inevitably become deaf during an attack due to the build up of fluid in the middle ear space, this is a temporary state of affairs and once the fluid has cleared the hearing will return to normal. It is extremely unlikely (although potentially possible) that any permanent damage will be done to the hearing as a result of an attack of acute otitis media.

The other worry that parents have is that their children are getting too many courses of antibiotics and that this will in some way interfere with their ability to combat infection in later life. Although in the ideal world it would obviously be better not to use antibiotics, each infection is an isolated and independent event and as long as the antibiotic course is completed, the infection will clear, and the antibiotic will pass out of the system. If there is no other treatable condition in the ears, nose or throat to prevent attacks, then it is better that the child should have antibiotics than the acute otitis media be untreated. There is no doubt that some infections are caused by viruses which do not respond to antibiotics but at present we have no easy means of identifying which are viral and which are not and the 'fail-safe' method is to use antibiotics for all attacks of acute otitis media. There is no specific treatment available to treat viral infections.

Acute otitis media is by far the commonest cause of earache in children. It does and can occur in adults although far less frequently. All that has been said about treatment, etc applies equally to adults and children.

Eustachian Tube Obstruction

I think we are all aware from time to time of having a blocked feeling in our ear and if this becomes permanent it can amount to actual pain or else can be extremely irritating.

The acute form of this ear pain can occur if we go flying (or

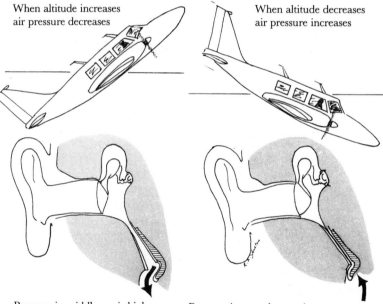

When altitude increases air pressure decreases

When altitude decreases air pressure increases

Pressure in middle ear is higher than in nasopharynx, and air escapes through Eustachian tube. Pressures are balanced automatically

Pressure in nasopharynx is higher than in middle ear. Because of flap value mechanism of Eustachian tube, it must be opened by deliberate action (e.g. swallowing) to balance pressures.

Note: When awake, we swallow once a minute; when asleep only once in 5 minutes
So when flying, particularly when descending, stay awake!

Fig. 6 The Eustachian tube in action

9

diving) with a cold. This is because the lining of the Eustachian tube swells up like the lining of the nose and completely blocks the tube. As the atmospheric pressure changes in the plane, the pressure in the middle ear does not and acute pain will be experienced. Some people are prone to this even if they have no cold and the only possible treatment is the judicious use of decongestant nose drops for an hour or two before flying.

In the chronic form of this problem the only treatment is the trial of a course of oral and nasal decongestants in an attempt to 'clear' the tube. In the really resistant group of patients, grommet tubes may need to be inserted. This will be discussed in detail in Chapter 7.

Trauma to the Ear

It has already been clearly stated that the skins of the ear and the ear drum have lots of very sensitive nerve endings. Any direct trauma to them can be exquisitely painful. It is a mistake to try and 'clean' your ears with orange sticks, cotton buds or knitting needles as you could perforate the ear drum or at least inflict pain on yourself.

The ear drum may be perforated in this way or in numerous other ways. A slap across the ear may force a sufficient column of air into the narrow canal to perforate the ear drum, as may landing on the side of your head when attempting to dive. Acute perforation of the drum in this manner will be momentarily very painful, may be associated with some bleeding and a feeling of deafness. The treatment is to keep the ear dry and consult your doctor as further damage may have occurred.

The Itchy Ear

This is a very common complaint and it is really a form of eczema (a skin disease) of the skin of the ear canal. It is called *otitis externa* (see also pp. 13-14). It used to be called 'Hong Kong ear' as it was frequently seen in people who went swimming in doubtfully clean water in hot, humid countries. The predominant symptom is that of a deep-seated itch but there may be actual pain and if the infected debris builds up in the ear canal then there will also be deafness and, not infrequently, discharge from the ear.

As the name of the condition suggests it is a disease of the external ear and as such does not produce any long-lasting damage to the ear from the hearing point of view. Having said that, it can be a particularly persistent and recurrent problem which is often resistant to treatment and can cause a lot of discomfort.

The important point for the treatment of otitis externa is to seek medical help sooner rather than later as once it has become chronic, recovery time will be prolonged. The other major aid to treatment is to keep the ear dry at all times. This involves keeping water out of the ears when swimming (better avoided altogether) and also when bathing, washing hair, etc. Sometimes in recurrent cases the treatment may require to be continued on a long-term preventative basis. Again, you should avoid 'itching' the ears with orange sticks etc., despite the temporary pleasure it may give!

Pain from other Areas

As can so often be the case in medicine, pain in one particular area does not necessarily mean that the problem lies in that area. Hence pain in the ear does not always mean ear disease. We can easily experience quite intense ear pain when the problem lies in our teeth, our sinuses or even some form of neuralgia. This is called *referred pain* and perhaps the classical example of this occurs not infrequently following a tonsillectomy operation. The child (or adult) may experience quite a severe ear pain on swallowing or eating, several days after surgery for their tonsils. This does not indicate ear disease but merely that one particular nerve (the glossopharyngeal nerve) has a very sensitive branch to the ear as well as a branch to the tonsil bed.

If pain in the ear persists for any length of time and is unexplained then it is important to seek medical advice.

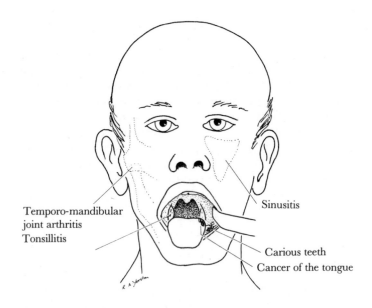

Fig. 7 Sources of referred pain in the ear

3. The Running Ear

The more correct term for this is the discharging ear, but either term can be used. It indicates the phenomenon of fluid coming from the ear and is often first identified by a telltale 'stain' on the pillow on wakening in the morning.

Perhaps one small misconception is worth mentioning. I am often told by patients, often mothers of children, that their ears or their child's ears 'run all the time'. On pursuing the matter further it turns out that the offending 'discharge' is, in fact, soft brown wax and this, of course, is quite normal and perfectly acceptable. There is a natural movement of wax out of the ear all the time as has already been mentioned.

Otitis Externa

As has already been mentioned, this condition is an eczema (skin disease) of the skin of the ear and the first sign may be pain or discharge from the ear: it is probably the commonest cause of discharging ears. The ear canal is quite a narrow passage and if the skin of the ear becomes infected from partially polluted water, with warmth encouraging the growth of organisms, then the ear canal will swell up inside, discharge, and often become painful. Nowadays, with increasing numbers of people holidaying in Mediterranean countries, the condition is understandably on the increase.

The best treatment is avoidance. If you have any tendency to eczema or dry skin elsewhere on your body, then it is advisable to either protect your ears with commercial ear plugs or cotton wool impregnated with simple vaseline. Alternatively, swimming with your head out of the water and avoiding diving is just as effective. Once the condition has started, medical treatment is required as although no damage will be done on a long-term basis, the condition will inevitably progress and become worse.

Otitis externa does not only occur, of course, in people swimming abroad. It can occur in anyone and particularly those who have a tendency to eczema or have dry, scaly skin. If you have these problems then you should make efforts to keep your ears dry at all times, be careful with hair sprays, try and clear dandruff and take note if the attacks are related to any changes in shampoos or even face make-up.

Treatment

The treatment of otitis externa is never easy. The basis of treatment is to keep the ears dry and eliminate any identifiable cause. Once this has been done, the use of antibiotic drops, with or without hydrocortisone, may be sufficient. Usually it is preferable to have a culture of the infected material so that the correct treatment can be given as sometimes people are actually allergic to some of the antibiotics in the drops. If the debris can be cleaned from the ear then an application of an antibiotic/hydrocortisone ointment to the skin of the ear may be sufficient to complete the cure.

'I had itchy ears when I was young but when I was in my twenties the itch got steadily worse. On consulting my GP, his solution was to syringe the ears to get rid of wax. This led to temporary relief but then I found that I was scratching the skin around the outer ear. By then I was sent to a specialist who diagnosed that (1) I produced more wax than the average person and that (2) I had outer-ear eczema. I used to try to poke the ears with a match stick and cotton wool. This only resulted in pushing the wax further into the ear, which resulted in real total deafness. Meanwhile the itch continued and the more I scratched the worse the eczema got, and weeping often occurred down the cheeks. Various specialists tried a selection of creams and even packing the ears twice a day for five days. Eventually I was given ear drops which resulted in a total cure; by this time I was in my early fifties. For me it has been a miracle.'

Wax in the Ear

There are a variety of ear drops available on the market for softening or dissolving wax in the ear canal. These are generally no more effective than simple olive oil drops and I have seen some quite nasty allergic reactions to wax solvents. In general terms, if you are one of these unfortunate people who tend to accumulate wax in their ears, then I would recommend the regular use of olive oil drops (say once per week) to keep the wax soft and allow nature's processes to move the wax out of the ear. Syringing of ears may be necessary but should be avoided if possible. The reason for this is that syringing seems to alter the natural process of wax movement and hence the intervals between visits for syringing become shorter and shorter.

If an ear discharges for any reason other than otitis externa, then it generally indicates a perforation of the ear drum. There are two common sites for perforations to be found (see Figures 8 and 9).

Anterior or Central Perforations

Anterior perforations are found in people who have had repeated attacks of acute otitis media. The ear drum becomes gradually weakened by repeated infections and ultimately it will break down and leave an anterior or a central perforation. This

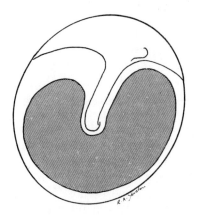

Fig. 8 Central, (non-marginal) perforation
of the tympanic membrane (ear drum)
A perforation within the shaded area, not extending to the
margin, is relatively safe, regardless of size.

indicates what is called tubo-tympanic disease as it is usually associated with people (often children) who get repeated upper respiratory tract infections, with the infection spreading up the Eustachian tube to the tympanum or middle ear space. These are looked upon as 'safe' ears as the infection will never spread beyond the ear and will not cause any damage to the ossicles. Usually these patients have intermittent episodes of discharge from the affected ear. There will be no pain and the discharge will often be quite profuse and sticky (mucoid). These episodes may occur in association with an upper respiratory infection or if the patient has been swimming without protecting the ear. The discharge will usually settle quickly with antibiotic treatment and the ear will remain dry until the next occasion. People either live with this problem and prevent episodes as much as possible by keeping their ear dry or else they have an ear drum graft operation (myringoplasty) to close the perforation. This is usually recommended if the problem is particularly recurrent. Being a graft operation there is no guarantee of success but in general terms approximately 80% of operations are successful.

Posterior or Attic Perforations

In contrast to anterior perforations, posterior or attic perforations are associated with persistent foul-smelling discharge from the affected ear. Again this is painless and because of this, people tend to live with the problem. They have often been to the doctor on one or two occasions and courses of antibiotics and/or ear drops have failed to help. The natural reaction is then to give up, as with no pain the problem does not seem worth fussing about. This is a mistake as the infection is due to attico-antral disease which means that the infection has spread from the middle ear itself into the ossicles and/or the surrounding mastoid bone. Once this has happened the infection is most unlikely to respond to antibiotics and will tend to slowly but inevitably spread through the bone. If this is allowed to persist over a long period of time then the infection may spread beyond the immediate bone to surrounding structures such as the brain or the facial nerve (which supplies

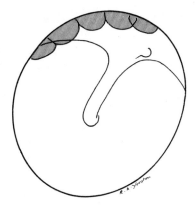

Fig. 9 Posterior or attic perforations of
the tympanic membrane (ear drum)

Perforations in the shaded areas, which extend to
the margin, are dangerous, even when quite
small

the muscles of our face). Very often the first bones to be affected
are the little ossicles and if these are damaged then a deafness will
be obvious. There may often also be bleeding associated with the
discharge and this again suggests a significant attico-antral
problem rather than a simple tubo-tympanic one.

Mastoid Surgery

As has already been suggested, antibiotics rarely resolve the
problem although they are worth trying in the early stages. The
only satisfactory way of treating infected bone is to remove the
involved bone surgically. The mastoid bone behind the ear is
exposed and, using a drill, the infected parts are removed
completely. This may involve removing an infected ossicle and
hence mastoid surgery does not, as a rule, improve the hearing.
The aim of surgery is to remove all infected bone so that the ear
will stop running and the ear will become safe from further
potential complications. It may be possible at a later date to go
back to re-operate on the ear to try and improve the hearing but
the primary object of the surgery is to stop the ear running and
prevent any complications. People who have had mastoid

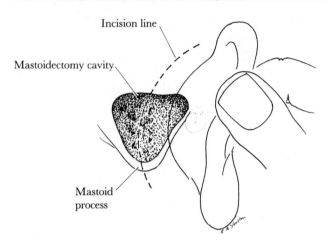

Fig. 10 Simple mastoidectomy

operations should continue to attend an ear, nose and throat specialist on a long-term basis as the cavity in the bone created by the surgery will require at least annual attention to avoid the excessive accumulation of wax and debris in what is a man-made artificial cavity.

4. Tinnitus

What is Tinnitus?

Tinnitus is difficult to define but it is basically the sensation of noises in the head. There are various degrees of tinnitus and in his autobiography, Mr Jack Ashley MP describes tinnitus as the head noises which 'plague' the sufferer, the ceaseless 'racket' which hinders concentration, prevents sleep and haunts the mental state of the sufferer.

How Common is Tinnitus?

This is a difficult question to answer as we have all experienced brief episodes of tinnitus at some time or another. The Institute of Hearing Research sent a questionnaire to a random sample of 6804 people in Cardiff, Glasgow, Nottingham and Southampton in 1979—1980. In the pre-pilot study, 39% of the people questioned claimed to have tinnitus but once they had been asked to exclude spontaneous tinnitus of less than 5 minutes duration and temporary sound-induced tinnitus, this figure dropped to 15—18% in the four cities. In the four populations sampled, tinnitus caused severe annoyance in 0.4-2.8% while a severe loss of ability to lead a normal life was reported by 0.4%. The percentage reporting tinnitus increased significantly with age and a history of exposure to noise. Tinnitus is, therefore, a very common problem and this fact alone often helps to reassure sufferers that at least they are not alone in their misery.

Types of Tinnitus

Tinnitus has already been described as a sensation of noises in the head. People's interpretations of the nature of these noises are often very varied and some of the common ones are:

- Low-pitched 'noise of the sea'

- High-pitched whistle

- Roaring of machinery

- Multiple sounds—together or separately

- Complex sounds

Many other descriptions are given and clearly seem to depend to a certain extent on the patient's imagination. The degree of loudness also varies a great deal and does not seem to relate specifically to the cause of the problem if this can be identified.

The age of the patient and the psychological state of the patient seem to be very significant.

Predisposing Factors

By far the commonest factor predisposing to tinnitus is age, and is usually associated with a high frequency sensori-neural (see p. 43) type of deafness so often encountered in the elderly. The second most common predisposing factor is a history of exposure to noise over a prolonged period of time. I think we all have experienced a temporary deafness with tinnitus after exposure to loud noise and this spontaneously resolves in a very short time. However, if this noise exposure persists over a prolonged period, permanent damage to the hearing will result and tinnitus will often accompany this.

There are other 'causes' of tinnitus that are worth mentioning although it is, I think, important to stress that in the vast majority of patients with tinnitus there is no identifiable cause (apart from deafness already mentioned). Otitis externa or even wax in the ear canal can cause tinnitus as can *all* pathological conditions of the middle and inner ear. Together with deafness, earache, discharging ear and dizziness, tinnitus is one of the symptoms of ear disease and usually offers little guidance to a doctor's diagnosis.

Tinnitus may be associated with a variety of diseases, the taking of certain drugs and the ingestion of some food and drink products. Common diseases associated with tinnitus are reduced thyroid function, raised blood pressure, diabetes and migraine. Efforts should, therefore, always be made to exclude these. The commonest drugs to cause or aggravate tinnitus are aspirin, indocid (for arthritis), quinine (for malaria and croup) and ventolin (for asthma). The commonest drinks to cause trouble have been found to be coffee and strong tea, tonic water, red wine and grain-based spirits (e.g. whisky, gin, vodka). The foods most commonly identified as a cause of tinnitus have been cheese and chocolate.

Although it is undoubtedly worth each individual sufferer considering all these points and perhaps experimenting with dietary change, it has to be said again that in the vast majority of patients the tinnitus will continue, as the cause of tinnitus has yet to be clearly identified.

Mechanism of Tinnitus

To doctors, specialists and research workers, tinnitus is a most tantalising subject. Although it is not in itself life-threatening, the amount of misery caused the world over is quite considerable. Sufferers often feel that because medical experts can so often offer no help they are in some way disinterested in the complaint and look upon it as a minor nuisance that is not worth bothering about. This is far from the case. The basic trouble is that to date, despite the expenditure of vast sums of money by researchers and drug companies, the mechanism of tinnitus remains unknown.

It is not even possible in any given patient to always identify the site or 'source' of the tinnitus. This may be from the outer ear, the middle ear, the cochlea, the nerve of hearing or even the central connections in the brain. I myself have seen patients with severe deafness and tinnitus in one ear. Complete surgical destruction of the cochlea and hence the hearing part of the ear, will render him or her completely deaf in that ear but they will almost always continue to experience their tinnitus just as if nothing had been done.

Until the mechanism of tinnitus is clearly defined, specific treatment will probably not be available.

Treatment of Tinnitus

Obviously the first step in treating tinnitus is to try and identify a specific cause and, if possible, cure the disease, treat the condition or avoid further aggravation such as noise, drugs, etc. It is, unfortunately, a fact of life that it is only in a very small minority of patients that this is a possibility.

Sufferers of tinnitus are sometimes very nervous people who feel that the tinnitus indicates something serious such as a brain tumour. Brain tumours *never* present just with tinnitus and, therefore, that worry must be forgotten. Tinnitus will often be worse when you are tired or anxious or just alone. This happens with everyone and the more you worry about it the worse it will become. People often are concerned that the noises will become worse and worse as they get older. This does not seem to be the case and in fact once you accept that you have to live with the problem, the intensity of the noises seems to lessen rather than increase.

It often helps to talk through your worries with other people, especially other sufferers. There are now tinnitus associations in all major cities and they do a huge job in uniting fellow sufferers and allowing them to share their problem with others who are equally or often worse afflicted.

For a few patients this is not enough and they desperately seek further help. There is no operation for tinnitus. Obviously if there is an identifiable cause, surgical correction may cure the tinnitus, although, as has been already suggested, this is certainly not guaranteed. There is no specific drug or medicine for tinnitus. Sometimes tranquillisers or sleeping pills may take the edge off things but they are only 'damping down' the effects rather than treating the real cause. Experiments into a variety of drugs continue but to date there is nothing available that gives any great hope for the future.

Tinnitus Maskers

People found by trial and error that if they went to sleep with the radio on or if they turned the radio slightly 'off' a station, the resultant noise tended to equalise their tinnitus and allowed them sufficient peace to get off to sleep. Some people still use this method on a clock radio system and it can be quite effective.

From this notion the idea of producing a noise, equal in loudness and if possible in frequency to the patient's tinnitus, developed. Small machines which look like hearing aids have now been developed for this very purpose and they are available through the National Health Service. Like so many machines they do not offer a total answer but they are of particular use if:

- the deafness is not excessive

- the tinnitus frequency can be reliably located

- the tinnitus can be completely masked by a band of noise at a low sensation level

Specialist ear, nose and throat clinics dealing with these problems are being set up and there is no doubt that some of the worst sufferers are being greatly helped by these tinnitus maskers.

One tinnitus sufferer describes the experience:

'I have had tinnitus for eleven years. It started as a slight buzzing in my right ear. At first I didn't pay too much attention to it, thinking it would go away, but instead it gradually got louder and began to pulse. Having never heard of such a thing before, I wondered if it was my imagination, or if I was becoming neurotic, and I was reluctant to talk about it to anyone. It was therefore a relief when I eventually discovered it was not "all in the mind" but that I was suffering from a recognised medical condition.

For a long while I felt very depressed. The noise in my head was insistent—it never stopped day or night—and I used to sit and listen to it and wonder how I was going to cope with it. Then I realised that this was the worst thing I could do and that I must try to divert my mind from my tinnitus. I started taking a real interest in my various activities and discovered that the more I became engrossed in them the less I thought about my tinnitus, so that it became more bearable and sometimes even less noticeable.

When a Tinnitus Self-Help Group was started in my area I joined it, and was amazed to discover how many people suffered from the same problem. It helped enormously to be able to talk to other people who heard unexplained noises in their heads and who understood what I was talking about. It didn't make my tinnitus any quieter, but it helped me to understand my problem better and to put it into perspective.

Now, eleven years on, I have more or less learned to live with my tinnitus. Some days are worse than others, and I would love to experience silence again—even for a little while. Being in a Self-Help Group, I now know that many people suffer more severe tinnitus than I do, but I have found that I can best cope by avoiding stress, trying to relax, and keeping myself occupied and interested in all I do.'

5. Deafness

Deafness is perhaps rather an emotive word as it sounds very final and complete. Those that work in this field prefer the term hearing handicap but as deafness is in such common usage I will continue to use this term.

Types of Deafness

It is very important to understand that there are two quite distinct types of deafness that can occur. This is important because, without an understanding of the different types, an appreciation of what can and what cannot be done to help is impossible. The two types of deafness are called *sensori-neural deafness* and *conductive deafness*.

Figure 11 shows a schematic drawing of the hearing part of the ear described in Chapter 1. If something goes wrong with this model central to the line separating the middle ear from the cochlea, i.e. something goes wrong with the cochlea (the nerve of hearing or the central connections), then obviously the patient's hearing will not be normal and deafness will result. This type of deafness is called a *sensori-neural deafness* and it is most commonly associated with the aging process. As a general rule there is no specific treatment to 'cure' sensori-neural deafness and our efforts have to be directed towards prevention and the use of hearing aids when and if required.

If something goes wrong with the ear external to the line separating the middle ear from the inner ear (Fig. 12) then a *conductive deafness* develops (see Chapter 7). As the name suggests, this means that something has gone wrong with the mechanism for conducting the sound from the outside air through the ear canal and middle ear to the cochlea. Again in general terms it is often possible to clear or treat this type of deafness and on many occasions completely restore the hearing to normal levels.

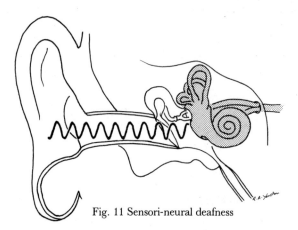

Fig. 11 Sensori-neural deafness

The sound wave traverses the outer and middle
ear normally, but the inner ear is unable to
perceive it because of disease in the cochlea
or the nerve pathways

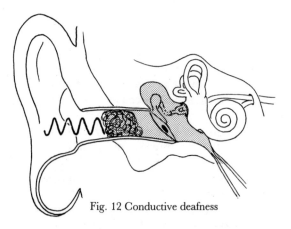

Fig. 12 Conductive deafness

Inner ear is intact and able to perceive sound, but
sound wave is prevented from reaching it by
e.g. wax, perforation, damage to ossicles etc.

Having defined the difference between sensori-neural and conductive deafness there is a third kind of deafness that can develop. This is called a *mixed deafness* and can occur in someone who already has a pre-existing sensori-neural deafness and then develops an obstructive or conductive deafness on top of that. It may, therefore, be possible to cure the conductive element of the deafness but, as there is a sensori-neural element to the deafness, it will not be possible to restore the hearing completely to normal.

Degrees of Deafness

How is the decision made that someone is deaf and how, once the decision has been made, is the degree of that deafness measured? Our hearing is, for all practical purposes, of most use to us for hearing the spoken word. It is, therefore, possible to test someone's hearing by doing simple voice tests. As a rule of thumb, if you can hear someone whispering from 4—6 feet from either ear then you are not effectively or significantly deaf. Poor progress at school is often put down to a possible deafness—often by the teacher and less often by the parents. This may, of course, be the case and it is absolutely vital that deafness should be excluded before any definite decisions are made regarding on-going education. It is, however, my experience that inattention is commoner than deafness and to convince the parents I will demonstrate by using the whispered voice test that the child's hearing is normal. It is important to block out the ear you are not testing and to cover the child's eyes with a piece of paper to make sure they are not lip-reading. It is often very impressive when the child hears the whispered words and the parents do not! Obviously, by using a variety of words it is possible to test different sounds and each ear can be tested separately.

Measurement of Deafness— Audiograms

The 'whispering' test is very effective but obviously it is rather crude and more accurate answers are required if there is any suspicion of a significant deafness. Hearing is measured using a machine called a pure tone audiometer and the results are produced on a graph which is called an audiogram (Figure 13).

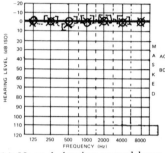

(a) Normal showing normal bone conduction and air conduction levels for both ears.

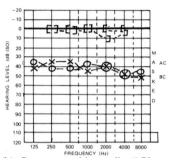

(b) Secretory otitis media ('Glue Ear') — showing bone conduction levels normal in both ears and air conduction levels at 30-40 dB in both ears, i.e. a conductive deafness.

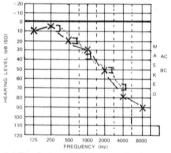

(c) Presbyacusis (left ear only shown for clarity normally both ears affected.) Bone conduction and air conduction levels equally affected and worse in the higher frequencies, i.e. a sensori-neural deafness.

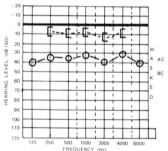

(d) Otosclerosis (of right ear). Bone conduction slightly reduced with air conduction levels at 40dB — typical findings in a young adult with otosclerosis.

Fig. 13 Typical audiograms

On the audiogram the intensity of the sound is plotted against its frequency. Most sounds are characterised by periodicity, i.e. repetitions that occur at the same rate over a period of time. One successive compression and rarefaction constitutes one cycle of a sound wave (Figure 14). The frequency of the sound is the number of cycles that occur in one second. Since 1960 the term hertz has been commonly substituted for cycles per second. This is in memory of a famous physicist called Heinrich Hertz and the abbreviation for hertz is Hz.

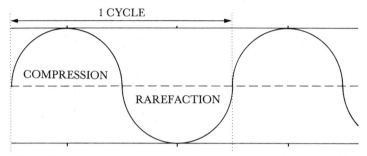

Fig. 14 Diagram of sound waves showing how one successive compression and rarefaction consititute one cycle.

The human ear has certain limitations in the sound frequencies it can be aware of and in a young adult this will range from 20—20 000 Hz. This is called the *audible range of frequencies*, but for practical purposes the ear is most sensitive to the frequencies from 500—8000 Hz. These levels coincide with the so-called speech frequencies and it is within this range that our hearing must be normal to reproduce and understand normal speech. The audiogram is, therefore, important in demonstrating the hearing levels between 500 and 8000 Hz. Speech is a very complex series of sounds but in simple terms vowels are low frequency sounds and consonants are high frequency sounds. Clarity of speech is heavily dependent on hearing consonants and if someone has a high frequency deafness they will have far more difficulty in discriminating speech than someone who has a low frequency deafness. This statement without vowels, 'sh.ps s..l .p th. F.rth' is fairly easily recognisable as 'ships sail up the Forth' while a similar statement '..e .e... .ea ..e...' with vowels and without consonants is far more difficult to decipher as being 'she sells sea shells'.

The commonest type of sensori-neural deafness is a high frequency one and this is why deaf people will always know if you are talking to them but will have difficulty in defining what you are actually saying due to their high frequency deafness failing to make out clear consonants.

The vertical axis on an audiogram measures the intensity of sound. The intensity of a sound wave refers to the strength of the particular vibration. The normal human ear is sensitive to a wide range of intensities. Sound intensity is measured as a ratio between power and pressure of sound and was named a bel after Alexander Graham Bell. The bel itself is too large a unit for practical purposes and it has been subdivided into ten parts called decibels (abbreviated dB). The least intensity corresponds to the minimum audible threshold of the ear (0 dB) and the highest intensity represents the point at which in the average person, the sound produces a sensation of pain (120 dB).

A pure tone audiometer is an electronic instrument for measuring an individual's hearing sensitivity. Measurements obtained with a pure tone audiometer are called hearing levels and are expressed in decibels (dB). These levels can be tested at various frequencies as described.

Impedance Audiometry or Tympanometry

Pure tone audiometry (as described above) is a *subjective* form of testing hearing as it requires the patient's co-operation. Impedance audiometry or tympanometry, as it is more commonly called, is an *objective* form of testing the compliance or movement of the ear drum and ossicular chain under conditions of changing ear pressure in the external meatus. This is an objective form of audiometry because it does not require the participation of the patient. It is of no use for measuring hearing levels but it is of great use in trying to determine the cause of conductive deafness in middle ear disease. It is most frequently used in detecting children who have secretory otitis media or 'glue ear'. If the middle ear is full of thick glue-like secretions then the Eustachian tube will be blocked. There will be a negative middle ear pressure and the compliance (or mobility) of the ear drum will be significantly reduced. Tympanometry is a quick, painless test and is very useful in diagnosing or distinguishing the cause of conductive deafness due to middle ear disease.

Distraction Audiometry for Testing Babies' Hearing

It is obviously not possible to do pure tone audiometry on a baby as, being a subjective test, there is no possible way to tell whether a baby is hearing a pure tone noise or not.

We are not born with the ability to speak. Speech is acquired in a way which is totally dependent on adequate hearing at all frequencies but particularly at the higher frequencies. For some reason that has never been scientifically explained, the first two years of life are vital for the acquisition of normal speech and language. It follows, therefore, that it is very important to be able to test a baby's hearing as, if there is some deafness, then it must either be treated or the baby must be supplied with appropriate hearing aids as early as possible.

Distraction audiometry is the method used to test a baby's hearing. The theory behind this form of testing is that if a baby hears normally then he or she will hear everyday domestic noises such as speech, music, rustling of paper, rattles, etc. Babies are naturally curious and if a noise with which they are familiar is presented to them they will always turn to identify the source of the noise. This response is not reliably demonstrable until they are able to hold their heads up unaided and hence distraction testing should not be considered until the baby is 6-7 months old. Attempts to demonstrate responses before this age are not to be encouraged as the results are quite unreliable and often may be misleading. For instance, if you clap your hands loudly close to a newborn baby he or she will often jump visibly. This in itself does not indicate that the baby has normal hearing and is called a startle response. Many babies with quite significant deafness will give a normal startle response and the technique is not recommended.

Carrying out the Test

To carry out distraction testing the requirements are a quiet room (preferably sound-proofed), two experienced testers and a baby 6-7 months old who is awake, not crying, not too hungry and not with a dirty nappy! There should be no visual distractions such as an older brother doing circuit training round the room and the parents and testers must have time and patience. The baby must sit centrally on a parent's knee, facing one of the testers who must distract the child visually by any appropriate method. The second tester must creep up behind the baby to one or other side, keeping behind the baby's field of vision. Using a variety of everyday sounds, the second tester will present the sounds to the baby 4-6 feet from the testing ear at low intensity. If the baby hears the sound then he or she will immediately turn towards the sound and the side at which the sound has been presented. If there is no response then it must be assumed that the sound has not been heard and the intensity of the particular sound must be increased until a response is obtained. By using a sound level meter or decibel meter, it will be possible to measure the level of sound at which the baby is responding on both sides.

In experienced hands distraction audiometry is a very reliable form of testing, and health visitors working from general practitioner health centres are especially trained in these techniques.

I think it is important to stress one or two points relating to testing baby's hearing. If the mother, who is usually in closest contact with the baby, feels that there may be a problem of deafness then it is vital that testing should be carried out not only until the tester is convinced that all is well but also until the mother is convinced. Parents often feel they are just being fussy and will tend to accept casual reassurance rather than reliable distraction testing. In other words, if there *are* doubts then the baby is deaf until proven otherwise. Equally, if a baby appears to fail a routine screening distraction test then this must not be ignored and forgotten or put off for another month.

Babies do not look deaf. They are almost always totally normal in every other respect and it is extremely difficult for testers and parents to believe that this beautiful bundle of joy is not responding normally to the testing. As has been stressed already, time is of the essence and delays will only tend to prolong the adequate acquisition of normal speech and language. An abnormal response must *not* be ignored.

Elective Response Audiometry

Once again distraction audiometry is a subjective test which requires, to a degree, the baby's co-operation. What is really needed is an objective test which is quick, simple and reliable and which can be performed within the first few days of life.

Babies are born in hospital or at home under medical supervision and a test at this stage would give excellent blanket screening and would mean that fewer babies with significant hearing problems would remain undetected until aged 2—3 as happens at present. At present brain stem evoked response audiometry (BERA) and electrocochleography (E Cog) are available. Both these are reliable electrical objective tests but E Cog has to be done under general anaesthesia and requires the insertion of a needle through the ear drum. BERA usually has to be done under sedation and is very time-consuming.

Clearly, neither of these tests is the answer at present, but there is no doubt in my mind that before long there will be available a safe and satisfactory means of testing a baby's hearing at birth. There are many more sophisticated types of hearing tests which are used to help in the diagnosis of particular problems. These are only available in specialised ENT hospital audiological departments. The science of audiology is a rapidly growing one and most large centres will have experts with a specific interest and skill in the use of the most sophisticated forms of audiometric assessment.

6. Sensori-Neural Deafness

Sensori-neural deafness (see Figure 11 Chapter 5) can be present at birth and it can be in only one ear (unilateral) or in both ears (bilateral). The hearing levels are not always the same in both ears so it is very important that they are tested independently in each ear. If there is a big difference between the hearing levels in the two ears, hearing tests can be misleading. If there is any suspicion that there is a difference between the two ears then it is important that the 'good' ear is eliminated from consideration by making a loud noise in it. This is called masking. If this is not done then the sound waves presented to the worse ear may be conducted through the bone of the skull and picked up by the good ear. Patients will be unaware of this transmission of sound waves and may respond as if they are hearing the sound in the bad ear and this may give false results.

Sensori-neural deafness may develop in one ear or both ears at any time from birth to old age. There are many causes and some of the more common ones will now be considered.

Causes of Sensori-Neural Deafness

On average, 1 in 1000 babies are born with significant bilateral sensori-neural deafness. Deafness becomes significant when the hearing levels in both ears are at 30 dB or more (averaged over the speech range of frequencies). The significance, of course, will depend on the frequency of the hearing loss as it has already been explained that high frequency loss is more significant than low frequency loss.

Hereditary Deafness

The actual cause of the deafness can be identified only in approximately half of the children born deaf. In some of these there is a strong family history of deafness. The mother, father, or both, or else grandparents or aunts and uncles, may have been deaf from a young age, often from birth. A family history of deafness that develops with aging is not associated with the birth of a child with significant deafness. If the family history is a strong one, the likely cause of the deafness is hereditary. Genetic experts will be able to look into this in more detail and will be prepared to give some sort of odds on future children of the same family being born with a similar deafness. In these families with inherited deafness, there are often associated defects which also 'run in the family'.

In the 50% of children in whom no cause can be identified for the deafness, there may be a dormant hereditary factor, that is one which has not previously appeared in either side of the family.

If the mother and father of these children both have what is called a *recessive gene* for deafness, then this may never have shown itself in the family. The union of these two recessive genes from the parents can produce significant deafness in their baby. At present we have no means of identifying these specific recessive genes but the assumption remains that this is the likeliest explanation for the cause of deafness in these babies in which no other cause can be identified. Perhaps it would not be a step forward if we were able to study our genetic make-up to the degree that we could anticipate these potential developments without being able to prevent them.

'When Sara was born she was an absolutely normal healthy baby — there was no sign of anything. Until she was a year or even 15 months old we didn't really notice anything wrong. When she started walking and didn't answer when we called, our natural reaction was to put it down to her being naughty—just not answering. This went on for long enough. She was slow in talking, but then that is something that varies so much. So everything was just normal as far as we were concerned , until it reached a stage when we realised there was more to it than just naughtiness and slowness. So we took her along to a specialist, who diagnosed that she was really profoundly hard of hearing, profoundly deaf, which was something that as a parent I just could not accept. Such a strange thing, to suddenly find that here you have someone who looks just everything, but there is something not quite right.

Sara would be four at this time. From an early age we encouraged her to be interested in books. We read the usual children's books to her, and sitting on our knees, watching us read and looking at the pictures, she got quite a bit out of that. To me books are a very important part of the whole life of hard-of-hearing children. Because I found her deafness hard to accept, I was continually testing: she would be upstairs and I would be calling and once she said 'Come up! I can't see what you're saying' — which proves how early she was aware of lip-reading.

When it was time for Sara to start school, we sent her to an ordinary school — I still didn't want to admit that she was deaf — but she didn't make any progress there. After a year we decided to send her to the hard-of-hearing school. The headmaster and teachers there were very, very good, the subjects were excellent, and she progressed normally through school, doing quite well in her exams, until it was time to leave; then it was a case of what to do next. She went for a year to a commercial college for typing, and she now has a excellent job with a large, well-known company.

She uses a hearing aid — she chose not to at school — but sometimes, when the girls at work are talking, they'll realise she's missed a point and say "Did you hear ...?" Then they carry on the conversation, treating her as normal and one of themselves.

When Sara was nine, our son Mark was born. Of course we were watching from day one, looking out for signs. The doctors all said such things never strike twice, but they did. At a much earlier stage than with Sara we realised that Mark had the same slowness at responding. We couldn't believe it — it was really just a nightmare. However we now knew what we were dealing with, and that we could cope.

Books played a large part in his early life, just as they had with Sara: Mark is still an avid reader. At the age of five he went to a small private school, and after two years to the same hard-of-hearing school as Sara. He decided and was encouraged to go to university, which meant that to get the necessary qualifications (the school was not geared for this) he had to go to a further education college. At college, of course, Mark found a big difference. Suddenly the lecturer's back would be turned, whereas at school the teachers had always made a point of facing the children, as we did at home. However, he progressed well, and went on to university, where he studied chemical engineering. After graduating, he joined a company, did research for a number of years, and is now working on computers.

Both Sara and Mark seem to be well satisfied with what they're doing. I feel that what they're doing is probably what they would have achieved with hearing.

Maybe their life would have been different — who knows? Nobody knows the path that they will be going along. From the point of view of education getting them to the stage of doing a worthwhile job, I think Sara and Mark have done as well as the majority of children. I feel proud at what they have achieved.'

Inheritance may well play a major part in the cause of deafness in babies. There are, however, other causes which can be identified and it is worth considering some of the more common conditions leading to the birth of a baby with permanent sensori-neural deafness.

Rubella (German Measles) Deafness

It has been known for a long time that the virus responsible for the disease of German measles (Rubella) can affect the developing ears and eyes of the baby when the mother is pregnant. If the mother develops German measles between the sixth and twelfth week of pregnancy (this may well be before she is actually aware that she *is* definitely pregnant) then there is approximately a 50% chance that her baby will be born either with some deafness or with some eye problems. There are blood tests available that can be done on both mother and baby (when born) that will demonstrate the presence of the German measles virus but this will only confirm the cause rather than offer any hope of a cure or even specific treatment.

German measles as a cause of deafness could be eliminated if all girls in their early teens accepted the vaccine that is freely available on the National Health Service against the Rubella virus.

There is no doubt that other infections or diseases that may affect the mother during pregnancy can, and undoubtedly do on occasions, cause deafness in the developing baby. These are not as easily or clearly identifiable as German measles and it is important to remember that 999 babies out of 1000 are born with normal hearing. Drugs are always potentially dangerous towards the developing baby and some may affect the hearing. Hence, whenever possible and sensible, it is better not to take drugs during pregnancy. Obviously your own doctor will be able to advise you on this matter.

Deafness and Prematurity

The ear may develop perfectly normally through the pregnancy but may then be damaged during the first few days or weeks of the baby's life. It is known that the cochlea is a very sensitive organ which can easily be permanently damaged, particularly by lack of oxygen and also by high levels of bilirubin in the baby's blood. Babies born prematurely are often 'blue' in colour due to lack of oxygen and they may require to be nursed in an incubator into which oxygen is fed. Some premature babies develop jaundice (yellow skin and eyes) due to the raised bilirubin levels in the immature blood system and this may require to be treated with phototherapy. Premature babies are now surviving more and more frequently due to the skills of doctors and nurses in neonatal special care units. Often these babies have very 'stormy' beginnings to life and there is no doubt that sometimes the cochlea suffers damage resulting in permanent sensori-neural deafness. Every person is different in their sensitivity to oxygen lack and to high bilirubin levels and it is not possible to quote levels at which the ear will definitely be damaged. Obviously as medical knowledge develops these problems should diminish and at the moment it is important that all babies born prematurely should be followed up carefully until it can be clearly shown that their hearing is entirely normal.

These then are some of the causes of deafness in babies that can be identified during pregnancy and the immediate post natal period. Sensori-neural deafness can also be acquired at any time during life and again some of the commoner causes will be considered.

Mumps, Measles and Meningitis Deafness

Once again it is important to point out that people are all different and not everyone who develops any of these three 'M's will develop sensori-neural deafness. However, we do know that there is a definite association between these conditions and deafness and hence awareness of the problem and, if possible, prevention of the condition is the rule.

Measles can cause deafness in two different ways. A child with measles can develop an acute inflammatory middle ear infection which may perforate the ear drum and cause a conductive deafness. This will be discussed later. The virus of measles can also affect the cochlea directly without middle ear problems and if this happens sensori-neural deafness will be the result. There is now freely available on the National Health Service a measles vaccine and if, like me, you saw these children permanently deafened by measles, I am sure you would ask your doctor to give your child the measles vaccine.

Mumps is a different problem as at present there is no available vaccine against mumps and as a general rule mumps is not as severe an infection as measles. Mumps cause painful swellings of the parotid salivary glands and most commonly affects both sides. It is common in children but it can, and does, occur in adults. In a small number of people who get mumps, the hearing may be damaged by direct action of the virus on the cochlea. It is impossible to identify who is going to be affected but as a general rule the chances of deafness increase directly in association with the severity of the mumps.

This mumps deafness is unusual in that it always affects only one ear. I have never met anyone with both ears affected and equally I have never heard of any satisfactory scientific explanation for this fact. It is indeed just as well that this is the case as the deafness of mumps is usually a very profound one. Only the most powerful of hearing aids could be used and even then the responses could be doubtful. One-sided deafness of mumps is often missed by the family as children do not seem to be aware of a one-sided change and it is my experience that the problem is often not noticed until the child is about school age. Perhaps he may be on the telephone to Granny and parents suddenly observe that he completely fails to hear in the 'other' ear. Or if he transfers the telephone to the deaf ear he thinks Granny has gone away. There is no treatment for this problem and, as it is only a one-sided problem, there are no long-term educational or social problems.

Meningitis can, of course, be an extremely serious infection which may be due to an identifiable bacterium or 'bug' or may again be due to a virus. A patient with meningitis may have a very stormy time in hospital and, particularly if they are young, the relief of their recovery and return home may well obscure the reality that their ears may have been damaged. The deafness of meningitis is usually on both sides and is most frequently a high frequency type of sensori-neural loss. Once again it must be stressed that there is no treatment for this deafness which is due to permanent damage to the cochlea and again it is impossible to anticipate which child is going to be affected by the deafness. For that reason, it is increasingly becoming accepted practice that all young children who have recovered from meningitis have their hearing checked at some time during their convalescence. The earlier the deafness is identified the sooner advice and management can be initiated. Hearing aids may be required and detailed hearing tests will be necessary.

Drugs causing sensori-neural deafness

There are a small number of drugs that can cause sensori-neural deafness but the list is relatively short and it is not common nowadays to become deaf as a result of drug therapy. Years ago when streptomycin was the only available antibiotic to treat tuberculosis, there were a significant number of people who lost some of their hearing at the expense of being cured of what could have been a fatal disease. Some people would accept that as a small price to pay but nowadays there are other drugs available for treating tuberculosis so that the problem has really been resolved.

The dangers of using *any* drugs in pregnancy has already been stressed but once again the list of drugs that can affect the developing ear is a short one. This then is not a major worry and the potentially toxic drugs are well identified. Doctors using these drugs will be aware of the problems and will carefully monitor the level of the drug in the blood to make sure it does not reach levels at which it could be toxic to the ear.

Noise-Induced Deafness

This is a very topical subject as in the last decade industrial noise-induced deafness has been recognised as a problem which, if proven, can be rewarded with compensation.

The cochlear part of the inner ear is a very sensitive structure and, if it is bombarded with loud sounds over a prolonged period of time, it will gradually become first temporarily and then permanently damaged. The part of the hearing range that is damaged in the early stages is at 4000 Hz and, as has already been explained, this is one of the important frequencies for the appreciation of the consonants of speech. It is also the frequency at which tinnitus is associated with the deafness and hence this often co-exists with the hearing problem. If the damage is prolonged, then gradually frequencies lower than 4000 Hz will be involved (i.e. 3000 Hz then 2000 Hz and finally 1000 Hz). The hearing loss will ultimately be very similar to that associated with old age and it is sometimes difficult to distinguish between the two.

Some causes

Industrial noise is a common cause. In this country the level above which a noise becomes dangerous is 90 dB (85 dB in the USA) and it is now obligatory for firms who have people working in noise levels above this threshold to supply proper ear protectors (ear 'plugs' are not adequate) and also to have safety officers appointed to try and ensure that these protectors are actually worn. The trouble with ear protectors is that they are very effective and when they are worn communication becomes virtually impossible. It is not human nature to cut oneself off from one's workmates and hence the average worker will not be very keen on wearing his or her ear protectors. If a firm supplies ear protectors and makes efforts to encourage the workers to use them then they will not be liable for compensation payments if the worker develops deafness. The commonest occupations associated at present with noise-induced deafness are boiler makers in the ship building industry and coopers in the brewing industry.

Other noise can, of course, cause deafness. *'Disco deafness'* is a well recognised entity. The noise level of an average discotheque can be as high as 120 dB and the people most likely to suffer are those running the discos as they are doing this on a regular basis. It is folly for them not to wear proper protection. People attending the occasional disco are not really at risk although if their hearing was tested immediately they left the disco they would definitely demonstrate a temporary deafness at 4000 Hz.

The present trend of the regular use of personal stereos is also potentially dangerous to the hearing if the volume is too loud. Those people who shoot regularly are also very much at risk—this can be either at a shooting range or out on the Scottish moors. Once again ear protectors should be obligatory but are often resisted as being antisocial and anticonversational.

As in so many things, every person will vary in their susceptibility to noise. Two people can be exposed to an identical noise for the same period of time and one may be unaffected while the other may develop classical noise-induced deafness. Once the deafness is permanent it is irreversible and if noise exposure continues then the deafness will be progressive in direct relationship to the level and frequency of the continued noise exposure. This is, in reality, a totally avoidable problem and with proper health education and the use of protectors, it should become a disability of the past.

Deafness of Aging

There is no treatment in medicine to prevent aging. Many parts of our body slowly degenerate with age and the ear is no exception. During the Vietnam war many post-mortem studies were carried out on American GI soldiers who had been killed. These showed that from about the age of 21 there were signs of degeneration in the cochlea when the ears were examined under a microscope. Again, as so often happens, there is a wide variation in the speed and age at which people's hearing tends to deteriorate. If there is a family history of relatively early deafness then this will tend to be passed on to the next generation but this is certainly not a hard and fast rule.

Once again the part of hearing that deteriorates first is the high frequency part. People with deafness of aging, which is called *presbyacusis*, will first notice difficulty in hearing female voices and children's voices and this will be particularly troublesome when they are in crowded rooms or at meetings or in church. The consonants of speech are high frequency sounds and when we speak we use less energy in producing consonants than we do vowels. Speech without consonants will be heard but as we have seen (p. 29) will be difficult to interpret. These difficulties in discriminating speech are well known to all people with an aging deafness and if you add the additional hazard of tinnitus, then the affliction becomes even more trying.

As hearing loss progresses, difficulty will be experienced with door bells, the telephone and ultimately with the television. It is common for the elderly to complain that the young of today do not speak clearly enough. In fact I doubt if this has changed over the years but, of course, with the loss of consonants, speech becomes indistinct and the easiest people to hear are not those who shout (this makes the vowels even louder) but those who make a conscious effort to enunciate their consonants clearly.

If you have started to develop deafness then little variations in hearing, which we all suffer from time to time, become much more significant as they will tip the hearing from a precariously acceptable level down to an unacceptable level. It is, therefore, common for people with the deafness of aging to find that minor fluctuations in hearing from catarrhal problems or from wax suddenly make them feel very deaf. They hope that clearance of catarrh or removal of wax will restore their hearing to normal. In fact there is no real treatment for sensori-neural deafness and this is a hard fact which has to be faced with realism and, often, with resignation.

Management of Sensori-Neural Deafness

At the moment there are no drugs or operations that will treat or improve sensori-neural deafness. You may read in magazines or newspapers of operations for nerve deafness but these reports are misleading and often upsetting to people who clutch at any possibility that their hearing may be improved. It is true that surgeons can now operate on people with nerve deafness but the operations are only to implant 'microchip' type hearing aids into the affected ears and are not appropriate to any of the sufferers of sensori-neural deafness. They are used at present for a tiny minority of the population who have had totally normal hearing and who suddenly become very profoundly deaf in both ears. Even in the case of these people the techniques are far from reliable and many of them revert to the use of more conventional types of hearing aids. These operations are of no value at all to children born with congenital deafness.

Avoidance of Sensori-Neural Deafness

The best way of treating deafness is to avoid it if possible. Vaccines against German measles, avoiding drugs in pregnancy, improving the care of the premature infant and awareness of the possibility of damage to the child's ears, are all important.

Efforts to reduce noise in the community are important, but if this is unavoidable then the diligent wearing of adequate ear protectors during exposure to noise will prevent noise-induced deafness. Cotton-wool in the ears or even ear plugs are inadequate, and recognised ear protectors are the only effective way of preventing noise-induced deafness in susceptible individuals.

As medical knowledge advances, hopefully some causes of sensori-neural deafness will be eliminated. There is, however, no treatment for aging and once deafness has become established to a significant degree, then the only treatment is the use of hearing aids. These are improving in their effectiveness and are discussed in detail in Chapter 8.

7. Conductive Deafness

As has been mentioned in Chapter 5, if something goes wrong with the ear external to the line (see Figure 12) separating the middle ear from the inner ear, then a conductive deafness develops.

To a doctor or an ear, nose and throat surgeon, the problem of conductive deafness presents a different challenge. In sensorineural deafness the challenge is to prevent the process if possible, diagnose it early and advise on hearing aids when needed. In conductive deafness there is always the chance that either medical treatment or surgery may be able to restore or at least improve the hearing. The reason for this is that in conductive deafness the nerve of hearing is normal and if the defect in the conducting mechanism is 'repaired' then normal hearing may be restored. The commoner causes of conductive deafness will be described and the available treatment possibilities discussed.

Congenital Conductive Deafness

Babies are sometimes born with abnormally shaped external ears, and often in association with this cosmetic deformity there may be an absent external ear canal or abnormal ossicles. In these circumstances, if the cochlea is normal, then it may be possible to operate and fashion a new ear canal or else replace or re-position the abnormal ossicles. This is very difficult surgery requiring a skilled surgeon using an operating microscope. If the condition exists only on one side (and if the other ear is normal) then attempts at surgical correction are not usually advised as the results of surgery are disappointing. Even at their best they will almost certainly not restore the hearing in the affected ear to a useful level. Often, in fact, the best that can be done in these circumstances is to fashion an ear canal which is large enough to take a hearing aid. If the condition is the same in both ears then surgery is worth attempting but it should not be done until the child is aged between 2 and 3. A hearing aid may be worn on a head band until the surgery has been done.

Secretory Otitis Media or 'Glue Ear'

This is by far the commonest cause of conductive deafness in children and it seems to be occurring with increasing frequency. It is in many ways a condition fascinating to doctors because its true cause is not fully understood. Like so many conditions in medicine where the cause is uncertain, there is no clearly agreed form of treatment and everyone has their own individual ideas.

The frequency of the condition is difficult to identify because it often varies, but probably at least one child in ten will develop the condition at some stage of their young lives. In America and all developed western countries the condition appears to be on the increase and the Americans have called it the 'language deprivation syndrome' when it occurs in the very young.

In this condition, deafness is due to the presence of fluid or secretions in the middle ear. This fluid prevents the ear drum from moving normally in response to air waves. I often liken the condition to filling a drum with water and trying to make it resonate.

There are two distinct groups of children with middle ear secretions. There are the group who develop insidious deafness without any complaints of pain in the ear or even catarrhal symptoms. They present most commonly between the ages of 4 and 8 and may often not be recognised until they go to school and have routine school hearing tests. The deafness is usually between 30-40 dB. As normal speech is at the level of approximately 50 dB, these children will hear satisfactorily in the one-to-one situation but will have difficulty if sitting at the back of the class or when there is a lot of background noise.

The other group of children are often in a younger age group. They suffer recurrent attacks of acute otitis media, with severe earache and frequent trips to the doctor for antibiotics and decongestants. The antibiotic will tend to 'sterilise' the infected fluid in the middle ear but the sterile fluid will remain in the ear and cause a significant hearing loss. These children will thus carry a 'sump' of fluid in their ears which is prone to re-infection every time they get a cold and will also give them a permanent 30-40 dB conductive deafness.

Diagnosis

Diagnosing secretory otitis media is not always easy. Parents or teachers may notice that the child is missing things. The child may either sit closer to the television or else he may turn up the volume. Comparison with brothers or sisters is often the first clue that all is not well. Screening tests of hearing are very important in the identification process. Health visitors at well baby clinics may identify the problem in babies under one year and obviously at this age it is very important to distinguish conductive deafness from a sensori-neural deafness. This can usually be done by using impedance audiometry (see p. 30).

Once children are older and able to co-operate then pure tone audiometry can be done. Routine school audiometric tests are done in most schools at the ages of 5, then 8 and finally at 13. These are most important as they will identity abnormal results which will then be reported to the parents and the GP (see Fig.13).

'Glue ear' can, therefore, be suspected from the audiometric results. Simpler tests such as whispered voice tests and tuning fork tests are very useful and are probably not employed enough. The appearance of the ear drum will often lead to a diagnosis although this is far from always the case. The 'classical' appearance of the ear drum in secretory otitis media has been described in at least thirteen different ways!

The cause of secretory otitis media is far from certain. In normal circumstances the secretions in the middle ear should drain away down the Eustachian tube into the throat and ultimately into the stomach. If the Eustachian tube is not functioning normally or is blocked then the secretions will collect in the middle ear. It seems that the root of the problem is associated with some malfunction of the Eustachian tube. Further than that no one really knows. Attempts have been made to blame allergies (including food allergies), swimming, abuse or over-use of antibiotics, plus many other imaginative ideas. The simple fact is that no one really knows and there has never been good evidence to support any of these theories.

Fairly recently a very good study was carried out in Bristol which seemed to show that adenoids, which lie at the lower end of the Eustachian tube (at the back of the nose), play a part in the Eustachian tube obstruction. They are, therefore, important when treatment is being considered.

Treatment

Treatment of secretory otitis media is difficult. Medical treatment with drugs such as decongestants is difficult to assess as it is known that 20% of children with secretory otitis media will recover spontaneously within six weeks of the diagnosis being made, i.e. the secretions will drain away down the Eustachian tube. In the 80% that do not recover, surgery is required and as the secretions are often very thick (like 'glue') they need to be sucked out of the middle ear through a myringotomy incision in the ear drum. If the adenoids are removed at the same time as the myringotomy is performed (see Figure 15) 80% of children will have no further trouble.

The question of when grommet tubes should be used remains slightly controversial. The Americans call grommet tubes ventilation tubes, and this is probably a good name as their purpose is to allow air into the middle ear and hence act as a temporary alternative to the malfunctioning Eustachian tube. I personally tend to reserve the use of grommet tubes for those children who have had their adenoids removed or else who have very small or absent adenoids (under the age of 2). Others will reserve their use for when the secretions are particularly thick, and yet others will insert them every time they do a myringotomy.

Grommet tubes remain in place for a variable time, related possibly to the degree of elasticity of the ear drum. When they 'come out' they will always migrate out of the ear (rather than into the middle ear) and will lie loose in the ear canal for a period of time before appearing at the outer end of the canal. They may be out within a few weeks or they may remain in place for over a

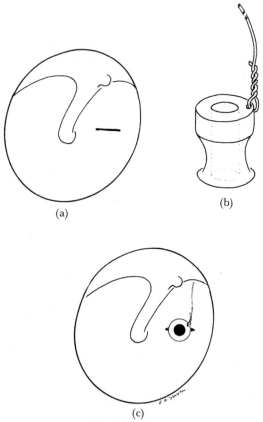

Fig. 15 Myringotomy
(a) incision line   (b) typical grommet (ventilation tube)
(c) grommet in position

year. Children with grommet tubes in their ear drums should avoid immersing their head in water, either in the bath or when swimming. The odd splash will make no difference but if water runs into the middle ear through the grommet, then infection may result and the ear may discharge infected fluid. Occasionally grommets may act as a foreign body in the ear and cause infection. In these circumstances they will need to be removed. Grommet tubes can be left in position for at least a year and often longer if they are causing no problems.

Adults can also develop Eustachian tube obstruction and this may or may not be associated with secretions in the middle ear. Perhaps the commonest occasion when blockage of the Eustachian tube is noticed is when flying at the same time as having a cold. Even although modern aircraft are pressurised this is never perfect and on taking off and landing there will changes in atmospheric pressure within the aeroplane (see Figure 6, Chapter 2). If the lining of the Eustachian tube is swollen because of a cold then the edges will stick together, the tube will block and a negative pressure will develop within the middle ear. This will at least produce a blocked feeling in the ear with some deafness and at worst produce acute earache with sometimes actual bleeding into the middle ear space. Some people seem to be much more prone to this problem than others. To avoid this unpleasant condition one should:

- avoid flying when you have a cold (if this is possible)
- suck a sweet or swallow madly during take-off and landing (the muscles of the palate open the Eustachian tube and moving the palate during swallowing or sucking will help to equalise pressures)
- use decongestant nose drops prior to flying in an attempt to prevent the lining of the Eustachian tube swelling.

Divers will, of course, experience identical problems which may be particularly severe if they descend too rapidly without equalising the pressures.

If secretions do collect in the ears then they may clear spontaneously. If not then myringotomy and grommet tube insertion will be required as there are no adenoids to remove in adults. Adenoids are present at birth and grow to their maximum size between the ages of 4 and 8. After this they start to shrink so that it is uncommon for a child over the age of 13 to have any adenoids.

Traumatic Perforation of the Ear Drum

This has already been mentioned in Chapter 2 as pain is always the predominant complaint. There will, however, always be some associated deafness and this will be of the conductive type.

The commonest cause of perforation of the tympanic membrane or ear drum is direct trauma. This may be due to poking pointed objects into the ear, syringing of the ear (very rarely), and can also occur as a result of explosions. There have been many large surveys of perforated ear drums reported from Northern Ireland.

The conductive deafness that results may be simply from perforation of the drum but can also occur if there is bleeding into the middle ear. Once the perforation heals this blood may collect and cause deafness in a way similar to the deafness of middle ear secretions. More severe trauma can also damage the ossicles in that they can be fractured or dislocated one from the other. All people who receive severe head injuries should have their hearing checked as injured ossicles can be replaced or re-positioned if the problem is identified early enough.

If damage to the ear is suspected then a doctor should be consulted. The treatment of a simple traumatic perforation is basically 'masterly inactivity' but nonetheless medical advice is important to exclude any possible complications. 90% to 95% of traumatically perforated ear drums will heal spontaneously within a few days and the hearing will return to normal at the same time. It is very important that the ear be kept completely dry during this healing process as water going through the perforation is liable to cause infection and prevent or delay healing. People should be advised not to swim and to protect their ears during bathing and hair washing.

Very occasionally the ear will not heal and a permanent perforation will be left. If this is the case then an operation can be performed to close the defect. This operation is called a *myringoplasty* and the perforation is repaired by using some fascia from the temporalis muscle which lies just above the ear. The fascia is used as a graft and like all graft operations, the success rate is not guaranteed although the results are generally good.

Infective Perforation of the Ear Drum

As has already been mentioned in Chapter 3 on the running ear, chronic otitis media is always associated with a perforation of the ear drum. When this occurs, there will always be an associated conductive deafness. The deafness may be due to the perforation alone or may be associated with damage to the ossicles. Infection in attico-antral disease can cause erosion of the ossicles and this will result in a significant conductive deafness.

The major purpose of surgery for chronic otitis media is to clear the infection and render the ear 'safe'. If the infection is not cleared from the bone, it can then spread into the head and can cause dangerous complications such as a brain abscess or meningitis. The associated deafness is a secondary consideration. However, if the ear is rendered 'safe and dry' then surgery to repair the ear drums and replace or re-position the ossicles can be carried out. This is delicate surgery carried out using an operating microscope and should only be undertaken by skilled ear surgeons. Any operation of this sort always carries a small risk of producing serious and permanent sensori-neural deafness and the patient should always be warned that this is a potential but unlikely complication of the operation.

The most recent advance in this kind of surgery has been the use of 'spare part' replacements. Ear drums and ossicles can be removed from bodies in the mortuary and stored in a special preservative fluid in the fridge. If, during surgery, it is found that the perforation of the ear drum is too large for repair or the ossicles are too badly damaged for re-positioning, then it is quite possible to replace the ear drum and/or ossicles by preserved specimens from the fridge. This is not transplant surgery as the replacements are not 'living' and hence there are no problems of rejection. Various silastic or other artificial replacements for the drum and/or ossicles have been invented and there is also a special 'glue' that can be used to try to stick everything together and reconstitute a mobile functioning ossicular chain. These are all exciting new advances in the field of ear surgery and have allowed surgeons to operate on ears to restore hearing as well as eradicate infection.

Otosclerosis

This is a condition which causes progressive conductive deafness, usually between the ages of 18 and 30. It is a hereditary

53

condition with a definite family history of deafness in 50% of cases. It occurs most commonly in women and the deafness often becomes worse in pregnancy. The conductive deafness is caused by the laying down of new bone around the bottom of the stapes or stirrup ossicle. This means that the stapes gradually becomes immobilised and hence the sound waves cease to be transmitted efficiently from the ear drum to the inner ear.

The patient will hear well with a hearing aid but as the deafness is progressive and the patient usually fairly young, surgery is most often advised. The original operation for this condition was called a fenestration operation when a large mastoid cavity was fashioned and the ossicular chain was by-passed. This operation was very successful but it was superseded in 1956 by a new operation called a *stapedectomy*. A young trainee American ear surgeon called Shea had the brilliant idea that the stapes could be removed and replaced by an artificial stapes made of plastic or, nowadays, silastic. This operation was so successful that it replaced the fenestration operation. There is at least an 80% chance of restoring the hearing entirely to normal but once again the patient must always be warned that there is a small (1%) chance of causing severe permanent sensori-neural deafness.

8. Hearing Aids

Hearing aids are machines which *amplify* sound but they can never replace the human ear. Having said that, however, they are vital to people with significant deafness and their efficiency and effectiveness are rapidly being developed. Hearing aids cannot, of course, be selective and the commonest complaint of hearing aid wearers is that they merely increase the noise level of sound but do not increase the clarity. This tends to make them annoying machines and many people fail to persevere with their hearing aids because of this annoyance factor. Deafness is often a gradual process and sufferers may be unaware that they have gradually ceased to hear certain sounds such as the traffic, the rustling of papers at breakfast time or the clanking of cutlery at meal times. If the aid is suddenly introduced then these sounds may become so dominant that they become almost unbearable and the aid is rejected. Patience and perseverance are required.

As has already been mentioned, speech consists of vowels and consonants. We use 65% of our speech energy in producing vowels and only the remaining 35% for the consonants. To discriminate speech content, the consonants are all-important and that is why the elderly have so much difficulty as they suffer from a high frequency (consonants) type of deafness. Their low frequency (vowels) hearing is usually very good and for this reason deaf people would prefer you to speak more distinctly rather than shout. Shouting will increase the total noise and the volume of the already loud vowels but will not go far in improving the consonants which are necessary for the clarity of the speech.

Having said all this, there is no doubt that hearing aids have a very important part to play in relieving the social isolation of those with increasing deafness.

Before hearing aids are considered, the ears should be examined by a doctor as there may be conditions that will be treatable. Occasionally there are conditions where a hearing aid may actually make matters worse. Simple removal of wax will never restore hearing to normal but it may be sufficient on occasions to make a hearing aid unnecessary.

People often think that if they start using a hearing aid they will become so dependent on it that their hearing will deteriorate and they will need stronger and stronger aids. There is absolutely no evidence to support this idea and, in fact, the best way to use a hearing aid is to put it on in the morning and wear it all day. This will make the aid part of life and it will not become a toy for occasional situations. The analogy with spectacles can be made. If you are short-sighted then you will wear your glasses all the time and not just when you think you are going to walk into things. Vision and hearing may well deteriorate slowly with age but aids to either are not going to hasten this process.

The importance of the early use of hearing aids in children with sensori-neural deafness has already been mentioned (Chapter 6). Two hearing aids must be worn during all waking hours and the constant input of sound throughout the day is vital. It is natural to think that if a child is deaf then there is no point in wasting time trying to speak to him or her. Exasperated parents may resort to gestures rather than persevering with the spoken word. It cannot be stressed too often that the future speech of a child with significant deafness depends on early diagnosis, good home counselling, and above all the diligent use of the best available aids backed by the constant input of sound. Aids are only machines but increasing sophistication is resulting in more and more effective instruments.

Types of Hearing Aids

The days of the National Health Service issuing a box and cord aid or a hearing trumpet have luckily gone and in the last few years, three different strengths of NHS aids have become available.

BE 10 series

The least powerful group are in the BE 10 series and these are ideal for an elderly person requiring help for hearing in church, meetings or crowded places. They are behind the ear aids (thus BE) and require to be fitted to an individually-made mould which is fashioned for the better hearing ear. People often find it difficult to understand why the aid should be fitted to the better ear but in the vast majority of patients, this is the most effective form of management. Sound waves bounce off walls, etc., and therefore will reach both ears on most occasions. Hearing aids work best when they are not turned up too loud and if they are fitted to the better ear they will produce maximum efficiency with minimum increase in the volume control knob.

BE 30 series

The middle series of NHS aids are the BE 30 series and they are definitely more powerful than the BE 10 series and may have to be supplied to people who are struggling with their original BE 10 aid. They are a very good series of aids but if the loss of hearing is only moderate then they will do no better than the BE 10 series.

BE 50 series

The most powerful behind the ear aids (sometimes called post-aural) are the BE 50 series. These are very powerful aids which can be individually adjusted to suit the particular patient's deafness and they have been a great advance for those with severe hearing loss.

Although there are only three different groups of NHS aids available, people have a very reasonable choice. The aids are made by firms on contract to the NHS and they are of a high standard. I have many patients who have a privately purchased commercial aid and a NHS aid, and a common remark is that they often find the NHS aid of more use than the expensive commercial one.

Commercial Hearing Aids

One of the big disadvantages of commercial hearing aids is that highly competitive advertising makes certain firms claim rather outrageous advantages for their particular model. This is unfortunate as there are available commercially a very wide range of extremely good and technically advanced aids. These are of particular value to school children with unusual types of congenitally acquired deafness. They will often require quite specific specialist type aids which could not be mass produced for the NHS. In its wisdom, the NHS does agree to purchase these specific aids for school children and for those in on-going academic education. Most of the aging public do not require these rather special aids and will function just as effectively with one from the BE 10 or BE 30 series.

'In the Ear' or Module Type Aids

These aids have been developed as a result of the use of the microchip, allowing continued miniaturisation of the hearing aid. These aids are a great advance and are the aids of the future. They are not available at the moment on the NHS (except for school children) but I have no doubt that in the not too distant future they will replace the behind the ear aid completely and will be available on the NHS. Their main advantages are:
- *Size* They are small enough for all the mechanisms to be contained in one case which is a little larger than the size of a normal mould.
- *Site* As it is so small it fits into the concave part of the ear and thus the sound waves are picked up by the ear itself rather than by a microphone behind the ear.
- *Specificity* As they have to be specially made for each individual so that they fit exactly into the ear, the working part of the aid can be specifically constructed to amplify only the worst affected frequencies. This means that they offer additional clarity of sound reproduction.

Radio Aids

These aids have made a huge difference to the management and development of the hearing of children with deafness. They are at present relatively bulky aids but their major advantage is that the teacher or parent wears a transmitter/microphone round their neck (or pinned to their clothes) and the sound waves are passed directly to the receiver which is worn by the child. The child's receiver has a switch which can allow him or her to receive only the radio transmitted waves or only the surrounding sounds or both. The aid can, therefore, be used as either a radio receiver (like a police walkie-talkie) or as a hearing aid or as both. This gives a hugely improved input in both the clarity and the volume of sound and has allowed children who would previously have had little chance of help to obtain good input of sound and hence develop good speech. These radio aids are very expensive and have the disadvantage of having to be charged every night. They have, however, revolutionised the teaching of deaf children in that more and more can go to their own community school and merely pass the transmitter/microphone to whichever teacher is taking them.

Home Aids

There is a huge range of aids available for use at home by the hard of hearing. Details of these can be obtained from the Royal National Institute for the Deaf (RNID) the address of which is listed at the end of the book. Loop systems can be fitted in homes or establishments and these allow sound to be picked up using the 'T' switch on the standard NHS aids. Louder door bells and telephone bells are helpful and additional flashing lights are available to help the profoundly deaf. Helpful advice will always be available from the nearest RNID centre and no one should ever be too embarrassed to ask for help.

Disadvantages of Hearing Aids

As has already been stated, hearing aids are only machines and they can never replace the wonders of the efficient normal ear. They can break down and wear out. They usually depend on some form of battery power and these can be of poor quality and will run down. A person wearing a powerful behind the ear aid every day will find the batteries will last only about three days.

A few people experience a very nasty complaint called *recruitment*. This occurs in a few individuals with sensori-neural deafness and manifests itself by the sufferer complaining that once sound reaches a certain loudness, it appears to be suddenly magnified to a point verging on pain. This is very difficult to do anything about as the critical level often seems to coincide with the degree of amplification required to make speech intelligible. Trials with altering the settings on the aid or using a different aid are the best ways of coping with recruitment.

'Squeaking' hearing aids are commonly heard and are as annoying to the wearer as they are to the normal hearing person. If an aid 'squeaks' continuously then it always means that the ear mould is not fitting properly and this must be replaced. An aid will, however, always 'squeak' when you cover it with your hand when it is switched on. This is due to a phenomenon called 'feedback' and this is normal. It is, in fact, quite a good way of testing to see if an aid is working or not.

Many elderly people have problems firstly understanding how their aid works and secondly managing to manipulate the increasingly fine control knobs and switches on the hearing aid. For this reason many aids very rapidly finish up in the back of a drawer as the person has been unable to cope with or understand the problems associated with this new machine. For this reason the medical profession is pushing very hard to encourage the appointment of more and more hearing therapists. These are specially trained technicians and advisers who will go out and visit the hard of hearing in their homes and offer help and support in the use of the aids and of the alternative home aids available. There is a great need in the community for more of this kind of help.

Cochlear Implants

Any chapter on hearing aids has to mention cochlear implants. These have been wrongly heralded in the non-medical press as the operation to cure sensori-neural deafness. Cochlear implants are minute hearing aids which are battery operated. They are so small that by an operative approach they can be implanted directly on to the surface of the inner ear. This diverts the sound waves straight to the cochlea and can give increased power for those who are very profoundly deaf.

At the moment they are not thought to be of use for those who have been born with profound deafness and have only been found to be of some help to those who have developed profound deafness after developing normal speech. They are not the answer to everyone's prayer but they may point the way towards future developments.

Lip-Reading

No discussion of aids for deafness sufferers can possibly be complete without mentioning lip-reading. All people with a hearing problem develop a natural ability to lip-read and they combine this skill with the sound that they obtain from their hearing aid. The more profound the deafness the more important lip-reading becomes. Lip-reading skills are most commonly acquired by self teaching. There are, however, classes available in most major areas where the skills of lip-reading are taught and addresses can be obtained from the RNID.

> 'I became deaf in my late teens after operations for double mastoid and brain abscess. With the help of my surgeon, my parents and friends, plus, of course, the resilience of youth, I soon learnt to accept my disability as a challenge and have been battling on ever since trying to play an active part in a normal hearing society.
>
> My hearing aid is my most treasured possession. Without it I hear little sound; with it, as if by MAGIC, I can follow speech and music. I used to be very musical, and I have retained my contralto voice, but I have, alas, lost the confidence to sing in public.
>
> Lip-reading throughout the years has been my life-line. We had no facilities in Perth around 1940 for lip-reading and I just persevered all day, every day, until I gained some proficiency in this art. With hearing aid, lip-reading ability and concentration I managed to cope.
>
> Over the years since those early days I have tried to help others come to terms with their disability; through helping them I've realised how fortunate *I* have been during my life-time. I have run classes in lip-reading with the backing of the local Education

Department. I have helped form clubs for the hard of hearing in several parts of Scotland and have formed many lasting friendships through the common bond of deafness.

In 1965 I moved up from the grass roots and became involved at National Executive level for many years with the work of the British Association of the Hard of Hearing. I am still working for the Association in different ways. The motto of BAHOH is ''Fellowship is Life''.

Through my normal hearing husband's career and interests I've had to take part by his side in public life—always with a little prayer on my lips ''Please help me to cope''.

Tinnitus and recruitment (see p.60) have plagued me all my hard-of-hearing lifetime and I have had many dark days. However, on reflection, my countless blessings and happy times far outnumber the shadows.

With wonderful advances being made in modern surgery and technology and a greater general public awareness of our needs becoming apparent, I look forward with confidence to a much brighter future for the many people like myself who have had the misfortune to acquire the Cinderella of all disabilities—DEAFNESS.'

Useful Addresses

TINNITUS

British Tinnitus Association
Royal National Institute for the Deaf
105 Gower Street
London
WC1E 6AH
Tel. 01-387 8033

DEAFNESS

Royal National Institute for the Deaf
105 Gower Street
London
WC1E 6AH
Tel. 01-387 8033

Royal National Institute for the Deaf (Scotland)
9 Clairmont Gardens
Glasgow
G3 7LW
Tel. 041-332 0343

Scottish Association for the Deaf
Moray House College
Holyrood Road
Edinburgh
EH8 8AQ
Tel. 031-556 8137

Scottish Centre for the Education of the Deaf
Moray House College
Holyrood Road
Edinburgh
EH8 8AQ
Tel. 031-556 8455

British Association of the Hard of Hearing
7/11 Armstrong Road
London
W3 7JL
Tel. 01-743 1110

National Deaf Children Society
45 Hereford Road
London
W2 5AH
Tel. 01-229 9272/4

National Deaf Children Society (East Scotland Region)
8b St Vincent Street
Edinburgh
EH3 6SH
Tel. 031-557 3757

Further Reading

TINNITUS

How to Cope with Tinnitus and Hearing Loss

R. Youngson
(Sheldon Press, 1986)

Tinnitus: facts, theories and treatments

D. McFadden
(National Academy Press, Washington D.C., 1982)

DEAFNESS

Deafness

J. Ballantine and J.A.M. Martin
(Churchill Livingstone, 4th edition, 1984)

Hearing Impairment: a guide for people with auditory handicaps and those concerned with their care and rehabilitation.

K. Lysons
(Woodhead-Faulkner, 1984)

How to Cope with Hearing Loss

K. Lysons
(Granada, 1980)

Deafness — Let's Face It

T. Sutcliffe
(RNID, 2nd edition, 1972)

THE DEAF CHILD

Our Deaf Children: into the 80's

F. Bloom
(Gresham Books, 2nd revised edition, 1978)

Educating Hearing-impaired Children in Ordinary and Special Schools	M. Reed (Open University Press, 1984)

THE DEAF ADULT

'The hard of hearing in Britain: are their needs being met?'	G. Rimmer

in

The Handicapped Person in the Community	D.M. Boswell and J.M. Wingrove (Tavistock Publications in association with the Open University Press, 1974)
Rehabilitation and Acquired Deafness	W.J Watts (Croom Helm, 1983)

SIGN LANGUAGE

Sign and Say. Books 1 and 2. These booklets contain the British (two-hand), American (one-hand) and deaf-blind manual alphabets, and photographs of about 800 British deaf signs.	RNID (RNID, 1981 and 1984)
Louder than Words	J. Hough (Great Ouse Press, 1983)

BIOGRAPHIES

Journey into Silence   J. Ashley
                                (Bodley Head, 1973)

Deafness: a personal account D. Wright
                                (Allen Lane, The Penguin
                                Press, 1969)

FICTION

In this Sign   J. Greenberg
                                (Gollancz, 1971)